Analyzing Emergency Department Medical Malpractice Cases

Patricia Iyer MSN RN LNCC
2014

The Pat Iyer Group
Fort Myers, FL

Analyzing Emergency Department Medical Malpractice Cases

Copyright 2014 Patricia Iyer. All rights reserved.

No part of this publication may be produced or transmitted in any form or by any means, mechanical or electronic, including photocopying and recording, or by any information storage and retrieval system, without permission in writing from the editors, with the exception of reviewers, who may quote brief passages.

Disclaimer: The Publisher and Author make no representation or warranties with respect to the accuracy or completeness of this work and specifically disclaim all warranties, including without limitation warranties of fitness for a specific purpose. No warranty shall be created or extended by sales or promotional materials. The advice and strategies of the author in this work may not be suitable for all situations. This work is sold with the understanding that the Publisher is not engaged in rendering legal, accounting or other professional services. Neither the Publisher nor the Author shall be liable for damages arising herefrom. The fact that an organization or website is referred to in this work as a citation or a potential source of further information does not mean that Author or Publisher endorse the information the organization or website may provide or recommendations it may make. Further, readers should be aware that internet websites and email addresses listed in this work may have changed or disappeared between the time this work was written and when it is read.

This product is for sale. Purchase a copy at www.legalnursebusiness.com.

Published by
The Pat Iyer Group
11205 Sparkleberry Drive
Fort Myers, FL 33913
908-391-7933
www.legalnursebusiness.com

Acknowledgements
The author appreciates the contributions of these emergency department professionals:

Jamie Byerly RN, BSN, CEN, CLNC, PHRN
Dean Dobkin MD, FACEP
Christine Macaulay MSN, RN

Cover design and layout by Zohaib Ahmad
Editorial support by Jill Lapinas and Jane Heron RN, BSN, MBA, LNCC

Legal nurse consultants: collect your valuable free ebooks at **www.legalnursebusiness.com**.

This book has been approved for 4 contact hours through an arrangement with Taylor College. The provider is approved by the California Board of Registered Nursing, provider number CEP-3285. CE credit is accepted in all states that require mandatory continuing education for relicensure. Call 1-800-743-4006 with CE questions. There will be a $15 fee, paid directly to the provider, if you want the CE certificate for 4 hours. See the form at the end of the book.

Table of Contents

About the Author 1

Introduction 3

Chapter 1: The Triage Process 5

Chapter 2: The Triage Role 13

Chapter 3: Triage Problems 19

Chapter 4: High Risk Triage 25

Chapter 5: The Wait 31

Chapter 6: Treatment Area Liability 41

Chapter 7: Investigation of an Emergency Department Medical Malpractice Claim 51

More Resources from Patricia Iyer 57

Book Evaluation Form 63

Contact Hour Form 64

About the Author

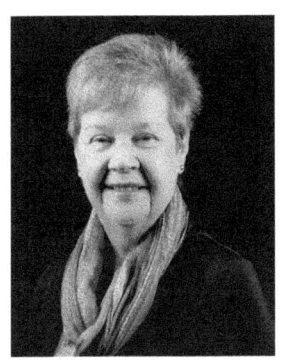

PATRICIA W. IYER, MSN RN LNCC

President, **The Pat Iyer Group** – education for legal nurse consultants at www.legalnursebusiness.com.

Patricia Iyer assists legal nurse consultants to skyrocket their businesses. Her coaching academy, LNCAcademyinc.com, provides education, support, encouragement and networking opportunities. She has been a legal nurse consultant since 1987 when she first began reviewing cases as an expert witness. She achieved national prominence through her texts and many contributions to the legal nurse consulting field. She was the chief editor of *Legal Nurse Consulting Principles and Practices, Second Edition*, the core curriculum for legal nurse consulting. She completed 5 years on the Board of Directors of the American Association of Legal Nurse Consultants including a term as president.

Pat was president of a legal nurse consulting business, Med League Support Services, Inc. from 1989 to 2015. She talked to attorneys about hundreds of emergency department claims before providing medical and nursing expert witnesses.

Reach her at patriciaiyer@gmail.com.

Analyzing Emergency Department Medical Malpractice Cases

Introduction

The emergency department (ED) is one of the highest risk areas of the hospital. (The old term "emergency room" implies that there is only one treatment room; this does not reflect the realities of a suite of rooms that make up the majority of today's EDs.)

Emergency department care may be an issue in a personal injury, medical malpractice or any case in which the patient required emergency services. Legal nurse consultants and attorneys need to understand how the ED staff functions. This knowledge is gained by consulting professional emergency care associations and emergency department expert witnesses. The Emergency Nurses Association was established specifically to define standards so that nurses would be aware of emergency nursing standards of care. The American College of Emergency Physicians provides guidance, standards and education for ED physicians.

There are several aspects of emergency department care that make it high risk for errors – the unpredictable flow of patients, the constant pressure to quickly assess and treat patients, the lack of a previous relationship with the patient, and the huge variety of conditions and the ages of the patients.

Legal nurse consultants and attorneys may encounter plaintiffs who are dissatisfied with emergency department care. The public is increasingly aware of emergency department quality of care issues. Demand for emergency department services is increasing. The public is paying attention to quality metrics or data. Overcrowding in the ED raises concerns about patient safety. Primary care physician shortages, reimbursement challenges and shrinking profit margins squeeze the staff of the ED even further. [1]

The emergency department is broadly divided into two areas: the reception area and the treatment area. The risk begins right at the front door when the patient walks in or is wheeled through the door to be triaged.

---

[1] Tocknell, M. Improving the ED, HealthLeaders, May 2013, 24.

Chapter 1: The Triage Process

What is triage

Nurses make up the largest category of ED healthcare professionals. They are expected to quickly sort patients upon their arrival into categories based on their complaints, and then assist in the diagnosis and treatment of conditions ranging from medical, surgical, pediatric, geriatric, psychiatric, obstetrical, and so on. Any age patient may come into the ED, from a newborn to a 100 plus year-old. Hours can go by with a light patient load, and then a busload of patients may arrive all at once. The stakes in the ED are high – to deliver the right type and amount of care in the face of unpredictable work flow.

Triage comes from the French word "trier" which means to sort or choose. Triage can be completed in a room, next to a stretcher or in the reception/waiting area. Triage is a process - not a place - in the ED. It is a process of sorting patients by their acuity (or degree of illness). This allows the triage person to identify those who need immediate care versus those who can safely wait. The purpose of the triage process is to get the right care to the patient in the proper amount of time.

Nurses are the professionals most often involved in performing triage. The triage nurse assigns each patient a triage severity score or category. There are two commonly used systems for categorizing patients based on three or five descriptors.

- The three category system uses the terms *emergent, urgent* or *non-urgent*.

- The five category system assigns a number from 1 through 5. Level 1 is the most life threatening and 5 is the least acute. The Emergency Nurses Association and American College of Emergency Physicians recommend the use of a five category system.

The process of triage

Although emergency departments are experimenting with how triage is accomplished, the process described below is a typical pattern.

Registration

A patient who arrives at the emergency department is usually greeted by a nurse or designated person. If that designated person is a unit secretary, not a nurse, the designated person will contact the nurse to alert the nurse of a patient's arrival. The usual first step in the care of any patient in the ED is registration. Basic information about the patient has to be collected (name, address, age, allergies) and an identification band placed on the patient.

If the patient arrives in a critically ill condition, registration is deferred until the patient can be stabilized or someone who knows the patient can provide that information. The patient may be known as "John Doe" or "Jane Doe" or some variation on those names until proper identification can be made.

The standard of care provides that a patient should be seen by a triage nurse within 10 minutes. If more than one patient arrives at the same time the triage nurse observes the patients and their complaints to see who may need medical treatment first.

After the patient is greeted, the nurse performs a rapid triage to rule out any life threatening conditions, before completing a more comprehensive triage. The complete triage process can take 1-5 minutes.

Nurses consider the ABCDs to determine the urgency of the patient's condition. Checking the ABCDs is done rapidly.

- "A" stands for *airway*. The triage nurse assesses whether the airway is clear from the mouth to the lungs.
- "B" stands for *breathing*. Nurses assess whether the person is breathing.
- "C" stands for *circulation*. If a pulse cannot be found, then there is no blood circulating. Emergency personnel may start rhythmic chest compressions (CPR). "C" also means to *check* for profuse bleeding which must be controlled.
- "D" stands for *disability*. It involves checking for injuries or symptoms.

During the comprehensive triage process, the nurse will ask key questions related to the patient's complaint. Some facilities use systems-based documentation forms. For example, as an attorney or legal nurse consultant, you may have reviewed medical records that contained an ED form focused on an orthopedic injury. All of the questions on the page are directed to the orthopedic history and symptoms. The physician's examination is also focused on an orthopedic injury. The triage nurse performs a limited assessment with specific questions related to an orthopedic condition, and the physician, nurse practitioner or physicians assistant takes a limited history and completes the physical examination. The focus of the assessment is to concentrate on why the patient is presenting for care.

Many facilities now use assessment protocols to guide the triage nurse in asking questions related to the common complaints that would bring a patient to the ED. Previously there were thick manuals that provided the protocols. Most facilities use computerized reference material and templates based upon common complaints so that it is easy for the nurse to select the complaint from a list and then use drop down menus to ask specific questions and individualize the care.

However, a focused assessment may result in the risk of missing other significant medical conditions that warrant immediate care. For example, ED staff members need to know some of the common diagnoses in certain populations. The ED staff has to understand the stated reasons for seeking care, but also be astute in picking up other serious concerns. The triage nurse may ask, "What brought you here today? What gives you the greatest concern?" Sometimes the triage nurse has to probe for the answers and more diligently question the patient to get to the root of the real emergency. The patient may have come in for a rash, but the real issue may be that he has run out of his medications and food and is living in a house without heat or air conditioning.

The nurse asks the patient why he came to the Emergency Department. This is called the *chief complaint*. The nurse will ask about past medical history, list medications and immunizations, personal safety at home (is anyone harming you at home?) and some other questions in reference to the complaint.

The triage nurse will take baseline vital signs: blood pressure, temperature, heart rate, respiratory rate, oxygen saturation using a pulse oximeter (which measures how much oxygen is in the blood) and assess the patient's pain. The goal is to quickly identify and begin treatment of emergent or Level 1 patients.

The triage nurse must notify the ED attending physician of concerns regarding patients who appear to be very ill. The triage nurse's duty is to recognize who needs to have further evaluation or immediate treatment.

Priority for ambulance patients

Another type of triage is to give priority to patients who arrive via ambulance. However, this system has been misused. Sometimes people who don't have the financial resources, a car, or anybody to bring them to the ED will call the ambulance because that is the only way to get there, but they may not have a serious condition. In some EDs, the charge nurse triages them. The charge nurse decides if the patient needs to receive immediate treatment and have a more comprehensive and focused assessment. Detailed triage information needs to be collected in a treatment room. The less ill patient may be sent to the reception area to be registered and triaged.

Documentation

The triage process is only complete when the information obtained during the assessment process has been fully documented. The nurse documents pertinent negatives, such as "denies nausea, vomiting, and diarrhea" - more commonly written as "no n/v/d". The symptoms the patient denies may be important pieces of information during the focused interview and used to assign the triage category and diagnose the patient's problem.

Communication of the triage category

The next step in the triage process is to communicate the patient's condition. The triage system conveys the degree of urgency for diagnosing and treating the patient. The way the communication is accomplished depends on whether the facility has a paper system or a computerized system. In a paper system the staff members use a medical record, which is the triage record. Many hospitals have a streamlined form that has areas where the triage nurse can document the chief complaint and then record all the essential data that needs to be collected. This includes medications, allergies, pain level, and other data.

The triage category, which is part of the communication system, is usually added to the chart so it's easily seen. The charge nurse and the ED attending physician may review the records. They look at the triage notes regarding the complaint, and review the vital signs and the data collected by the triage nurse. They might re-evaluate the triage category of some patients. A patient who has been put in the treatment area might be moved to the waiting area.

When there is a computerized triage system, the triage nurse enters the pertinent patient data including the patient complaint, the vital signs, the medical history, allergies or surgeries. Then the triage nurse will document the category or severity: Level 1, 2, 3, and so on. Anyone who has access to the computer will be able to view the triage level. All key people know who has come to the emergency department and can review the data about the patient.

Chapter 2: The Triage Role

Preparation for the triage role

Some facilities require the ED nurse to have prior experience in medical surgical or critical care nursing. However, with the current nursing shortage, there have been some modifications. At a minimum, the nurse should have an in-depth orientation with content and clinical experiences that would assure the nurse has the baseline knowledge that he or she would need.

After working in the ED for at least six months and receiving more education, the nurse should be sufficiently prepared for the triage role. The nurse should receive instruction about triage guidelines. Validation of the nurse's skills is typically performed by observing the nurse in action to verify he or she is able to accurately perform specific critical skills. This validation is done by another experienced triage nurse.

When only a registered nurse will do

Nurse practitioners, physicians and physician assistants may perform triage but typically a registered nurse completes the process. Registered nurses are educated in two, three or four year nursing programs. Licensed practical nurses (LPNs) have one year of nursing education.

When I was asked by a hospital to do an evaluation or an audit of their ED records, I found some instances where LPNs were doing triage. One of my recommendations was to not put the LPN in that position. Triage needs to be done by an RN. LPNs do not have the knowledge base to perform triage and should not do so. The LPN is not licensed to assess patients, but is expected to assist the registered nurse in performing tasks and collecting data. In the treatment area, LPNs may perform some tasks that are within their scope of practice such as administering oral medications like Tylenol.

Qualities of the triage nurse

The triage nurse should have these qualities:

- Ability to rapidly establish rapport with patients
- Ability to soothe frightened people
- Knowledge base to ask the right questions
- Analytical skill to sort through data to focus on the pertinent signs and symptoms
- Critical thinking skills
- Patient assessment skills
- Ability to be calm and decisive
- Ability to multitask
- Ability to document the appropriate data
- Knowledge of how to mobilize the department's resources for critically ill patients

The triage nurse should be a very skilled person who can ask the appropriate questions to determine patient acuity. Additionally, the triage nurse should be able to follow protocols which are designed, reviewed and revised on a regular basis by the medical director and the nurse leader - be that a nurse manager or a nurse director.

Demands of the triage role

Frequently there is only one triage nurse. The nurse has to know all the norms for various age groups. Patients of all ages may arrive in the emergency department. Severity of illness ranges from the patient who comes in with minor complaints to the person who is critically ill. The patient's complaints may be common or very rare. The triage nurse has to know what questions to ask to elicit the important details of the history and symptoms.

The triage role is mentally and physically taxing. The nurse may be constantly on the go, moving people and pulling people on and off stretchers or out of cars. The space is often inadequate for what the nurse needs to do. The emergency department is frequently very noisy, crowded, and overwhelming. The triage nurse's job involves making quick decisions about the seriousness of each patient's condition. When the decisions are wrong, or a patient's condition worsens unnoticed, serious outcomes may occur.

There are a lot of interruptions in the triage nurse's work flow. The nurse may be seeing people coming in and acknowledging them. But at the same time the nurse may be involved in interviewing somebody and has to stop to assess a new patient to make sure he or she is not presenting with an emergent problem.

Electronic medical records may add to the distractions. The nurse has to maintain eye contact with the patient while inputting information into a computer. Studies have shown that patients feel less significant if the healthcare provider stares at the screen instead of looking at the patient.

The triage nurse's job involves an incredible amount of multitasking with constant interruptions. The nurse has to have skilled clinical judgment based on a wide variety of knowledge and experience.

Role of unlicensed personnel in triage

A lot of hospitals use the registration staff as greeters in the reception area and give them a script of what they should say. If someone comes in with chest pain, for example, the greeter's script should direct her to get the triage nurse. This use of personnel also tries to balance the triage nurse's activities of interviewing patients and collecting their information with the greeter's ability to quickly acknowledge people who are coming into the ED.

Unlicensed assistant personnel – EMTs, paramedics, registrars, medical assistants, any type of aide or greeters – may not do an assessment. Sometimes hospitals wrongfully ask the unlicensed assistive personnel, such as medical assistants or registration personnel, to collect initial information about the patient's complaints. That is substandard and not consistent with the standards of the Emergency

Nursing Association or The Joint Commission, which accredits many facilities. Neither licensed practical nurses nor unlicensed assistive personnel are trained to perform assessments and assign triage acuity.

It's the registered nurse who has to analyze and assess that data to determine how sick the patient is.

Some hospitals are using unlicensed assistive personnel to help support the nurse. This may be appealing because of cost savings, but the registered nurse needs to supervise the unlicensed assistive personnel. The danger is that the unlicensed personnel might work outside of their scope of practice without even realizing it.

Chapter 3: Triage Problems

When the triage nurse or treatment area is overloaded

The work intensity can suddenly spike in the ED. A patient arrives in cardiac arrest and needs to be resuscitated. A patient suffers a major trauma after falling through a roof. An infant is gasping for breath because of croup. What happens if all of these patients arrive simultaneously?

It is the triage nurse who has to be very assertive, knowledgeable and comfortable with the role of expediting patient care. The triage nurse also has to be able to acknowledge, "I'm one person. I can't handle this alone and I need to get immediate help," or "We're overwhelmed and something may happen because we can't get to these patients who are in need of triage."

All hospitals have to have a backup plan; the plan applies not only to triage but also whenever there are more patients than can be comfortably managed. For example, there may be one or two ED doctors. Is there a plan for when the doctor becomes overwhelmed? Can the doctor call another doctor in? A large teaching hospital with residents has more resources than community hospitals do. A community hospital may have one doctor working during evening hours or two doctors working or on call during the high volume hours. They have to have a backup plan that also applies to the triage nurse. In some instances, the ED may need to notify rescue squads to stop transporting patients to the ED and divert them to other locations.

When no one is doing triage

A lot of hospitals have protocols for when the triage nurse is overwhelmed and cannot get to patients in a timely fashion. The triage nurse might be able to say, "What's your problem, what are you here for" but the nurse can't do the more detailed focus in a timely manner. The triage nurse has a responsibility to ask for help from the charge nurse to get more resources to manage the influx. Usually the solution is to call people in from home, but it takes time to make the calls and for the off duty staff to arrive at the emergency department.

Every emergency department should have a staff member assigned to monitor the reception/waiting area. This person may be a security guard, a registration person, a greeter, or a hospital volunteer.

> In *Henry Jones, individually and as representative of the Estate of Janell Jones v. Medical Center of Southeast Texas LP, et al*, Janell Jones was fifty-seven years-old when she underwent heart surgery. She was discharged six days later. Four days after discharge, she returned to the hospital because she was having chest pain. When she arrived at the emergency department, three nurses had to be paged before anyone could assist her into the waiting room. She was unattended in the waiting room for ten to twenty minutes despite being in cardiac arrest. She died in the emergency department. The plaintiff and defendants argued over what the autopsy showed as the cause of death. The plaintiff also alleged that the cardiothoracic surgeon misinterpreted the reason for an elevated heart rate seen on an EKG on the day of

discharge from the hospital after cardiac surgery. The jury found the cardiothoracic surgeon to be 25% negligent and the hospital to be 75% at fault. They awarded $4,510,000. Post trial motions were pending. [2]

In this case, the triage system broke down. The fact that three nurses had to be paged implied that no one was immediately available to perform triage. There was a delay in assessing and treating a critically ill patient.

When my husband and I took our adult son to the emergency department because he was having trouble breathing, there was one person (a clerk) at the desk. She asked why my son was there. We said he was having trouble breathing. She then returned to collecting insurance information from another patient. It was a half hour before our son was taken into the treatment area to be assessed. I could feel our anxiety levels rise the longer we waited. A nurse appeared only when we became insistent.

When a nurse friend of mine developed laryngeal spasms, her friends took her to a large inner city emergency department, where there was a glass window and metal tray for collecting slips of paper recording the patient's chief complaints. My friend wrote that her chief problem was "can't breathe". She waited 15 minutes and no one ever approached the window. A patient standing outside told her the name

---

[2] Henry Jones, individ. and as representative of the Estate of Janell Jones v. Medical Center of Southeast Texas LP et al, Jefferson County, (Tx) District Court, Case No. D-186,807. Reported in Laska, L. (Ed), Medical Malpractice Verdicts, Settlements and Experts, October 2013, page 14.

of a different ED where she would get faster attention. When she got in a cab, she found out the cab driver did not know where the other hospital's ED was located. After he dropped her off at the wrong corner, he drove around the block and came back to take her to the ED entrance. There she was promptly triaged and treated. Fortunately, the spasms stopped without ill effect.

If the triage nurse is with a patient or is not at the triage area, the patient should ask the first hospital employee he sees for assistance. If there is a phone present in the reception/waiting area and no one is available, the patient can pick up the phone and dial the operator and advise her he or she is in the emergency department and needs medical assistance.

When a disaster strikes

A trainload of passengers may arrive after a railway derailment, and they all need to be assessed and treated. Emergency departments should have disaster plans to deal with mass casualty events. When a disaster plan is activated it defines or includes the triaging protocols that apply when a group of people arrive at the emergency room at one time.

During a disaster, the ED staff may temporarily send somebody to the waiting room, or use other parts of the hospital to treat patients, such as the clinic or post anesthesia care unit. The ED may also declare it is *on divert* which means that ambulances are not permitted to bring any more patients in. This does not stop patients from going to the ED in cars. If it's a true disaster there are disaster plans required; there are disaster codes called, and a whole plan for carrying out care.

Disaster triage is different than ED triage in that the staff is trying to just make sure the people who can be saved get treatment immediately. If somebody comes in with a fatal wound, the staff may determine that no treatment is needed because he's not going to survive. Disasters test and strain the resources of the healthcare facility.

Chapter 4: High Risk Triage

Consider some of the reasons why plaintiffs end up filing lawsuits against emergency room nurses and physicians. One of the categories of allegations is failure to recognize or diagnose a problem or a delay in treatment of that problem. The following are some of the red flag issues.

"Worst headache of my life"

Most ED nurses are very concerned if a patient says, "I have the worst headache of my life." Those words alone should lead the staff to immediately take a patient to the treatment area. The symptom may represent some type of hemorrhage in the brain or impending neurological problem that needs immediate attention.

Severe pain

Another serious concern for nurses is the sudden onset of severe pain associated with symptoms of nausea, vomiting or chest pain. This also could be caused by a kidney stone if the patient has severe flank pain. The Joint Commission requires the healthcare staff to assess the pain level of any patient presenting to any healthcare institution. The pain has to be quantified on a scale. The most commonly used scale rates pain as a number from zero to ten, with ten being the worst possible pain. Patients who are unable to assign a number may be able to point to a drawing of a face that represents their pain. This is the FACES pain score. Hospitals may utilize different pain rating systems from those described above. Patients with severe pain need immediate attention.

Substance abusers

Emergency department personnel encounter patients with chronic pain. Staff may suspect they came to the emergency department seeking pain medication. These patients are a high risk for missed diagnoses because the staff may overlook medical conditions that are causing the pain. They may unfairly label the patient. The term "drug seekers" is a pejorative term at least partially rooted in the frustration that may build up in the ED staff when they encounter these patients. An ED physician took this feeling one step further and ended up being sued.

> In *Mayhew v Madison,* a thirty-year-old woman went to the ED because she had generalized pelvic pain, a vaginal discharge and a concern that she could be pregnant. Dr. Brent Madison ordered a blood test which showed the patient had barbiturates in her blood. Ms. Mayhew had no explanation for this. Dr. Madison found her condition to be normal. After he discharged her without a diagnosis or treatment, he learned she had obtained several prescriptions for narcotics. He called the police to report a suspicion that the patient was engaged in unlawful drug-seeking behavior. The police arrested her and charged her with unlawfully seeking drugs at the hospital. She was jailed, and then released after charges were dismissed. Ms. Mayhew filed suit against Dr. Madison. She alleged he was negligent in calling the police, in divulging personal information to them, and that she was suffering from endometriosis. She had surgery several weeks later.

The plaintiff pointed to Dr. Madison's own history of having his license suspended for substance abuse, and that he received a DUI after his license was fully restored. Dr. Madison claimed that his examination and treatment was proper and the phone call to the police was not part of the treatment. His defense was the plaintiff had only a malicious prosecution claim. The jury returned a $125,000 verdict. [3]

The plaintiff's investigation of Dr. Madison certainly yielded useful information. I suspect the defense counsel attempted to keep this information from the jury. Legal nurse consultants and attorneys may find out information about healthcare professionals by making inquiries with the appropriate licensing board. Check this link to reach the Professional License Verification Databases at **http://www.clearhq.org/resources/license_verification.htm**.

Pregnancy

Pregnant women experiencing abnormal symptoms such as pain and contractions constitute emergencies. Patients who might deliver in the emergency room may be having frequent and prolonged contractions. As a rule, ED staff transfer these patients to the hospital's labor and delivery (L&D) suite (if it has one) as quickly as possible. If a pregnant woman presents with a bloody show, ruptured amniotic fluid, or a fetal foot or hand

---

[3] Mayhew v Madison, Carroll County, KY Circuit Court, Case No. 10-66. Reported in Laska, L. (Ed) Medical Malpractice Verdicts, Settlements and Experts, October 2013, page 9.

sticking out, that requires immediate delivery in the ED.

For example, there was a young girl who didn't tell the ED staff she was pregnant. She said she'd never had sex, but in a few minutes the triage nurse was able to get information that indicated she was probably pregnant. The triage nurse's colleagues were skeptical about why the triage nurse took the patient right into the treatment room until the patient got onto the GYN table and the staff saw the baby's head was visible.

OB patients are high risk. When the staff is in doubt, the triage category should be of highest acuity. Often pregnant women have to be partly screened for the doctor. If no emergent issues are identified, the staff will send her to the labor and delivery (L&D) area to be assessed and monitored by trained L&D nurses. The triage nurse has to be astute in determining the safest way to transport that patient.

- Does the patient need to be transported by a nurse?
- Could something emergent occur during the transfer to the L&D department?
- Is this a routine complaint so that it will be safe to transport her via a wheelchair with only unlicensed assistive personnel?

Delays due to under triaging

The golden rule is if in doubt, the triage nurse should assign a higher triage category to a patient. For example, if a triage nurse cannot say, "I feel comfortable that this patient is a Level 3", she should identify the patient as the higher acuity Level 2. The nurse has to be confident about the conclusions based on data collected from the patient.

Chapter 5: The Wait

What comes next after triage: the wait

Most legal nurse consultants and attorneys have heard of patients who had a delay in ED treatment. The patient was triaged, sent to the waiting room, and then waited and waited and waited. Two questions arise:

1. Was the person appropriately triaged based on the complaints? Was there a delay in treatment given the severity of the symptoms?
2. How long should the patient have to wait for treatment? Was there a standard for how frequently the patient should have been assessed or how long should the patient should have expected to wait in the waiting room?

Factors that affect waiting time

How long is too long to wait? How long should a patient wait before getting up and walking out of the emergency department to seek care elsewhere? A lot of considerations go into a question like this. It is not possible to arrive at a precise mathematical calculation by trying to figure how many doctors and nurses were present and how many patients were waiting to be seen. The factors that affect wait time include:

- The number and mix of ED staff on duty
- The time of day
- The number of patients in the treatment area
- The condition of the patients in the treatment area
- If the department is on divert

- The number of patients who are boarding (waiting for a hospital bed)
- The number of open ED beds available for patients to be seen
- The location of the ED, with longer waits in urban areas than in nonurban areas
- The volume of annual visits to the ED, with longer waits associated with EDs who handled 50,000 or more visits per year [4]

The National Center for Health Statistics found that from 2003 to 2009, the mean wait time in U.S. EDs increased 25% from 46.5 minutes to 58.1 minutes. [5]

Use of protocols for waiting patients

The staff may follow protocols to administer some treatment while the patient is waiting for a more detailed assessment. Protocols define interventions such as administering medications to control fever to keep the patient comfortable or analgesics to treat pain. The nurse may follow protocols like initiating laboratory tests or ordering x-rays. The protocols have been approved by the medical director. The physicians and nurses determine the protocols for certain complaints that they know are common in the population served by the ED. The protocol provides standing orders for a certain complaint. For example, a patient who comes in with an ankle injury will probably need an x-ray of the ankle. If the patient is a child

---

[4] Wait Time for Treatment in Hospital Emergency Departments: 2009, NCHS Data Brief, No. 102, August 2012
http://www.cdc.gov/nchs/data/databriefs/db102.htm

[5] Id

presenting with a fever, there are usually Tylenol or Advil orders in place.

The use of protocols is consistent with the trend to encourage more independent decision making so that ED nurses are initiating some of the treatment based on the protocols instead of waiting for the physician to be available to order those tests or prescribe treatment.

There might be unlicensed assistive personnel helping the nurses and physicians. The ED's protocol may permit the unlicensed assistive personnel to draw the labs, do an EKG or escort the patient to x-ray. Any lab results are documented so when the doctor sees the patient he or she has more up to date information to better provide a medical screening, diagnosis and treatment.

Reassessment

Many EDs have created the expectation that emergency department nurses should reassess patients waiting in the reception/waiting area every hour unless the facility has a protocol stating otherwise. The ED triage nurse needs to reassess patients in the waiting room based on their level of acuity. A high acuity emergency patient would rarely be left out in the waiting room unless the patient was incorrectly triaged. An acuity Level 2 patient should begin receiving treatment as soon as possible. The nurses just might need a couple of minutes to make space for the seriously ill patient to receive care.

Most hospitals have reassessment policies. They shouldn't be waiting for attention for hours without being reassessed. The use of a camera in the reception area provides a way to monitor patients who are waiting, but does not replace reassessment procedures.

Patients also have an obligation to let the nurse know if they have a change in how they are feeling. Patient complaints can change and symptoms can worsen. If this occurs they must notify the triage nurse immediately that their symptoms are worsening or they think they may have had a change in their condition. Some reasons to notify the triage nurse might be difficulty in breathing, shortness of breath, chest pain, increasing pain, dizziness or feeling like he or she might pass out.

Patients should not hesitate to be insistent on attention if they feel worse, although this puts a big responsibility on patients who may not be in any condition to be assertive in getting attention. Requests for attention may not be successful. While waiting for my husband to be treated, I sat in an ED waiting room near a woman who rocked, clutched her abdomen, moaned and cried for over an hour. She had no success in getting treatment any faster.

Fast track

Some facilities use a fast track system. This is a way to identify patients who are non-urgent such as those who came in for a minor sprain or a minor fracture. The fast track system separates them from the critical treatment area where there's a lot of intense care being delivered and resources are very scarce while the staff take care of seriously ill patients. Some facilities set up fast track systems to rapidly move the patient from entry into the facility to discharge or hospital admission.

The fast track system often uses two registered nurses — one who is there to first meet and greet the patient within two to five minutes and one who does a more extensive assessment. The first nurse follows a quick process to identify the non-urgent patients. While doing that he or she must look at the patient's chief complaint and simultaneously determine whether the patient requires immediate care or can wait safely for more assessment by the second triage nurse. Once that decision has been made the nurse will log the patient in with a name and date of birth. Then the second triage nurse or nurses become involved. Many of these departments have three or four nurses backing up the nurses doing the initial decision-making about the entry of the patient into the system. The second nurse will perform a more detailed but focused assessment.

Leaving without treatment

Although ED staff members try to avoid it from happening, patients do walk out of EDs without being treated. Patients obviously have a right to leave if they want to. However, it may be a very high risk decision because the patient's condition has not been diagnosed or treated.

Emergency department personnel know that longer wait times will lessen opportunities to provide medical care to those coming through the ED doors. Inevitably, some people will leave without being treated. There is no solid evidence to show the patients who walk out are low acuity and may safely leave. In fact, the symptoms and urgency for treatment of these patients often elude ED staff; they are the "LWBS," the patients who "Left Without Being Seen".

Patients who are already in the treatment area are undergoing the process that will provide them with the care they need. They should stay. It may take a long time, but if they are under evaluation and treatment, leaving is a bad idea. Patients who leave after being triaged because they are tired of waiting may have a rude awakening if they go to another ED. They will start from scratch in the next ED.

Many EDs are working on expediting the process of moving patients more quickly into the treatment area. They are concerned about patient safety. Triage is not medical treatment; it's not medical screening. The nurse is obligated to encourage the patient to stay. The patients should be told it would be best for them to wait. They should understand the risks if they do leave and don't get treatment. And if they still choose to leave because they're tired of waiting, the nurse needs to inform the physician. The safest procedure is for the nurse to always inform the ED attending physician that a patient wants to leave so that the doctor can determine if he or she needs to speak with the patient about the risks of leaving without being seen.

If a patient does not speak English, the triage nurse needs to get an interpreter so that the person fully understands. Patients should receive information about the risks of leaving the ED in their primary language instead of the nurse's primary language. The need to communicate in a language the patient understands applies to all aspects of ED care.

A (Leaving) Against Medical Advice form needs to be signed when patient announce they are leaving. The patient must be able to say, "I understand and I know the risk and I'm leaving anyway."

Many times patients do not announce they are leaving. They may decide they are going to another ED or back home. The nurse may discover the patient is not there when the nurse calls the patient's name to do further data collection or reassessment or when it's time to bring the patient back into the treatment area. The nurse needs to make a diligent effort to locate the patient. The patient might have gone to the men's room or the ladies' room or to get snacks, especially if he or she does not have a really serious condition. Sometimes other patients in the waiting room will report that the patient left.

The nurse needs to document in the medical record when the nurse first discovered the patient was no longer in the waiting room. The nurse should record what actions were taken to find that patient such as, "Called the patient's name three times and there was no answer", and record the different times that he or she called for the patient.

Boarding patients - a different kind of waiting

A growing problem in almost every emergency department is "boarding" patients. The decision is made to admit the patient but there is no bed available inside the hospital. So the patient waits – is "boarded" – in the emergency department. Sometimes these patients are boarded for over a day. They require medical and nurse care. The emergency staff attends to them while less acute, less severely ill patients wait in the waiting room. In some settings, the medical surgical nurses or intensive care unit nurses take care of these patients in the ED.

The boarders tie up emergency department stretchers, thereby reducing the available resources for other patients. The beautiful, state-of-the-art, 28-bed emergency department may have 20 people waiting to be admitted. That leaves eight beds for ED patients. There may also be several patients in wheelchairs in the hallway.

> In *Gelene Salter, etc v. The University of Chicago Medical Center et al*, a young woman went to the emergency department because of a severe headache. She received pain medication and was sent home. She returned later the same day with the same symptoms. The physician recognized she was likely suffering from a malfunction of a shunt that had been inserted to drain excess cerebral spinal fluid. Surgery was scheduled for 4 days later. She was kept in the hospital's emergency department while she waited for surgery. The day prior to the surgery, the patient suffered a brain stem herniation due to fluid buildup, which caused severe and permanent brain damage. She was in a coma for a year before she died. The plaintiff alleged a failure to recognize that the intracranial pressure in her brain, which was five times higher than normal, required immediate intervention. The suit initially included the hospital and the physicians involved in the woman's care, but the physicians were dismissed from the suit. The plaintiff claimed that the surgeon who was scheduled to perform the surgery was

overbooked and there was a lack of communication between doctors, leading to a delay in treating the decedent. A $4 million settlement was reached. [6]

A four day wait in the emergency department is unusually long. These facts raise questions about the communication that occurred, or should have occurred, regarding the duration of the boarding and the type of care provided to monitor Ms. Salter's condition while in the ED.

An alternative to the traditional triage model

Many EDs keep careful statistics about the volume of patients and the number of people who leave without being seen or treated, or refuse to wait. The quest to improve efficiency led staff of the Cambridge Health Alliance in Massachusetts to rearrange the triage and assessment process. They first installed "patient partners" or non-clinicians who greet the patient and do a mini-registration to get the patient's name and chief complaint. The patient is then taken through a rapid assessment by a physician assistant or physician.

The nurse may perform the triage while the physician is simultaneously evaluating the patient. These innovations resulted in the median total length of the ED stay dropping from 220 minutes to less than 140 minutes. The number of patients who left without being

---

[6] Gelene Salter, etc v. The University of Chicago Medical Center, et al, Cook County, IL, Circuit Court, Case No. 08L010221. Reported in Laska, L. (Ed.) Medical Malpractice Verdicts, Settlements and Experts, July 2013, page 8.

seen dropped from over 4% of the total volume to consistently below .05%. The time from the entry through the ED door and the first physician evaluation averaged less than nine minutes. [7] Contrast this to the statistic cited earlier of a mean wait time of 58.1 minutes according to data from the National Center for Health Statistics. What an improvement!

---

[7] Jim Molpus, Emergency Department Efficiency, HealthLeaders, December 2013, pages 57-59.

Chapter 6: Treatment Area Liability

Once the patient is taken "into the back" for treatment, a new set of responsibilities emerge. The healthcare providers are responsible for diagnosing and treating conditions, communicating with primary care physicians and consultants, and making decisions about "disposition" – where should the patient go:

- Admission to the hospital
- Home
- Return to a nursing home
- Transfer to another hospital

Treatment area risks are high. The condition of the patient could deteriorate requiring rapid recognition of serious changes and quick intervention. The patient's food, fluid and elimination needs require attention. I once spent 8 hours with my mother in the ED and had to repeatedly ask people for a cup so I could get her water. Then I had to search for the only functioning sink in the ED.

Communication issues arise due to language barriers, distractions and changes in personnel from shift to shift or from one department to another. The risk of administering treatment to the wrong patient is high because of the constant turnover of patients and the need to move patients to different locations in the ED and other departments or a patient's inability to confirm his identity. The need to rapidly move patients through the ED ("production pressure") to prevent or relieve overcrowding increases the risk of missing something or making errors.

EMTALA requirements

The Emergency Medical Treatment and Active Labor Act requires that any patient who comes to a hospital's dedicated ED with what he or she believes to be an emergency medical condition be given a medical screening exam. In fact, the patient does not have to enter the ED to be considered as having arrived at the hospital. The patient could be within 250 yards of the hospital, on a sidewalk or in a parking lot and be considered to be seeking emergency services.

The emergency medical condition is one where a patient presents with acute symptoms of sufficient severity that in the absence of immediate medical attention could reasonably be expected to seriously jeopardize the patient's health or body functions, or cause serious dysfunction of any body organ or part. It also covers women coming to the ED in active labor. [8]

The ED has an obligation to the patient regardless of the person's ability to pay. The medical screening exam may be performed by a physician or other healthcare provider, such as a nurse, as long as the facility defines who may perform the exam, the medical functions the non-physician provider may perform and the provider follows his or her professional scope of practice. The exam should reasonably determine if an emergency condition exists, and include the necessary diagnostic testing. [9]

---

[8] Sally Austin, What does EMTALA mean to you? Nursing 2011, June 2011, pages 55-59.

[9] Id

Next, the staff needs to determine if they have the resources to treat the patient's condition. The ED is required to maintain a list of on-call physicians in various specialty areas. If the patient needs care from a specialist who does not meet his or her obligation to see the patient and no one else is available, the name and address of the on-call physician who failed to respond must be documented in the patient's transfer record. Failing to document this information may result in Centers for Medicare and Medicaid Services citations and fines against the ED physician, hospital and on-call physician. [10]

If the ED staff is not able to provide the appropriate level of care, they are obligated to stabilize the patient and transfer the patient to a facility that is able to meet the patient's needs. The receiving hospital must be capable of providing the services the patient needs, and the benefits of the transfer must outweigh the risks. The receiving hospital may not refuse to accept the patient because of an inability to pay for care. The patient's vital signs and a discharge summary need to be documented prior to transfer. The patient is to be sent to the receiving hospital with diagnostic studies, medical records, and the transfer documentation. [11]

EMTALA creates a framework for ED staff to help avoid fines and lawsuits. Some of the liability risks this law highlights include:

- Refusal to treat a patient who has no ability to

---

[10] Id

[11] Id

pay for care
- Failure to perform a medical screening exam
- Failure to transfer a patient to a facility capable of providing a higher level of care when needed

Common allegations

Many things can lead to an emergency department patient seeking a plaintiff attorney. These are some of the common allegations.

1. *Failure to recognize signs and symptoms of the worst possible problem may result in missed diagnoses.* For example, failure to diagnose a myocardial infarction (confusing it with gastrointestinal symptoms) may result in delays in treatment and death. Hospitals are expected to follow policies, procedures and protocols developed by nationally recognized organizations like the American Heart Association.

   A three-month-old infant was taken to the ED because she had a fever of 103°. The ED physician diagnosed her with a middle ear infection and discharged her with a prescription for amoxicillin. There was no documentation of which ear the infection was in, or what was seen in the ear. The next day the child was pale, cool to touch and lethargic. Her parents took her to the pediatrician's office, and then to another hospital, where she was diagnosed with pneumococcal meningitis, hypoxic brain injury and hydrocephalus. She was hospitalized for a month and ultimately died almost two years later from respiratory complications. Her parents sued the emergency department physician, alleging that he should have ordered a blood count and urinalysis to rule out the possibility of bacteremia and meningitis and that he should have scheduled a follow up evaluation 24-48 hours after the first visit. The defendants claimed that the physician was not negligent and could not have reasonably foreseen the child's clinical course. The defendants specifically claimed the bacteremia and meningitis developed after the child left the ED and the strain of pneumococcus responsible for the problem was resistant to amoxicillin. The jury returned a verdict of $1.7 million. [12]

2. *Failure by the nurse to communicate the patient's condition in a timely manner to the ED attending physician is a major source of liability.* The nurse has the training and is licensed to screen the patient for emergent conditions that need immediate treatment. There are risks when nurses fail to communicate the patient's condition in a timely way and the patient's condition then deteriorates.

3. *Failure to adequately assess patients while they are in the waiting room and failure to reassess the patient may occur.* The patient's condition may worsen in the waiting room. The frequency of reassessment needs to be defined in the triage guidelines set by the hospital's clinical leadership.

---

[12] Takacs v. Reading Hospital and Medical Center, Berks County (PA), Common Pleas Court, Case No. 09-9629. Reported in Laska, L. (Ed) Medical Malpractice Verdicts, Settlements and Experts, September 2013, page 9.

4. *Delays in treatment may be due to overcrowding.* Treatment may be hurried, superficial and not address important conditions or symptoms. This increases the risk of missed diagnoses.

5. *Failure to anticipate safety needs of the patient causes liability.* For example, not transferring a patient appropriately is an issue. The patient may fall while trying to get out of a wheelchair onto a stretcher or fall off a stretcher trying to get to the bathroom when a nurse is not available to help.

6. *Injuring the patient during diagnosis or treatment causes liability.* There is a wide range of interventions that can injure patients, from intravenous therapy insertion errors, medication errors, puncturing the lung during a tube insertion, removing cervical collars before the patient's neck has been tested for fractures, and so on.

   In an Ohio case, a 42-year-old man was taken to the ED after he became confused and disoriented after not taking his schizophrenia medications. He became increasingly aggressive and refused care. At one point he was forcibly restrained so he could be given a sedative. After he was admitted to the hospital and the sedation wore off, the staff discovered he could not move his legs and had limited use of his arms and hands. A neck fracture at C5-6 was diagnosed. He had surgery but did not recover function. The plaintiff alleged negligence in the way he was restrained. The defendant asserted the healthcare providers had acted properly. The jury returned a verdict of $2,866,521.35. A post trial motion was pending. [13]

7. *Failure by the nurse to notify the ED attending physician of abnormal test results in a timely way may result in injury.* For example, an abnormal EKG done while the patient is waiting to be seen by the physician should be immediately shown to the physician. The nurse is obligated to document her interventions, which are "EKG done, given to the doctor", and to document what orders the doctor gave.

Common Defenses

1. *It did not happen here.* The defense is based on disputing the facts. The defense will assert that the injury occurred either before or after the ED care. A careful timeline of events may prove this to be true.

A 68-year-old man went to the ED with a chainsaw laceration of his left knee. He alleged that a month after this visit, he developed a severe infection in the knee, which required surgery, intravenous antibiotics and physical therapy. The plaintiff claimed that antibiotics should have been given at the time of the ED visit and that a partial cut to the quadriceps tendon was not diagnosed. Defense asserted that

---

[13] Michael Dillon v. OhioHealth Corp, Franklin County (OH) Court of Common Pleas, Case No. 10CV009220 reported in Laska, L. (Ed), Medical Malpractice Verdicts, Settlements and Experts, August 2013, page 10.

there was no indication for prescribing antibiotics, and that if the plaintiff had an infection at the time of the ED visit, it would have been evident at that time, rather than when it was diagnosed a month later. The defendant claimed the wound was cleaned and examined before being closed.

The defendant claimed that the plaintiff was given a special staple remover to take to his primary care physician which was intended to minimize tissue damage during staple removal. The defendant also claimed the plaintiff was instructed to follow up with his physician in 12-14 days for reevaluation and staple removal. The plaintiff removed his own staples after three days and never followed up with his primary care physician. The plaintiff claimed that when he was handed the staple remover, a nurse or physicians assistant told him he could remove the staples himself. A defense verdict was returned. [14]

2. *The actions of the plaintiff contributed to the injury.* This defense may be particularly effective if the plaintiff acted in a reckless way and caused his injuries. The standard of care to be delivered to a patient injured by his own actions should be the same whether the patient caused injury to himself through his own actions or the patient was blameless. The jury has a tendency to

---

[14] William Warnick v. UPMC Passavant, Allegheny County (PA), Court of Common Appeals, Case No. GD-11-012960, reported in Laska, L. (Ed), Medical Malpractice Verdicts, Settlements and Experts, September 2013, pages 10-11

harshly judge people who make poor decisions. The case described in the first common defense is a good illustration of a patient whose actions (removing his staples and not following up with his physician) may have contributed to his poor result. It is very hard to believe an ED staff member would tell a patient to remove his own staples.

3. *Hindsight bias.* The filing of a suit always occurs after we know the end of the story or what happened to the patient. The defense argues that in hindsight, it is perfectly clear what the symptoms should have suggested as a diagnosis and what treatment should have been rendered. The defendants did not have the benefit of hindsight.

4. *The ED staff used judgment.* The staff members have the right to use medical or nursing judgment in treating the patient. The outcome of care cannot be predicted; a patient may be injured even if care is appropriately rendered based on the judgment of the provider.

5. *The patient withheld information that would have been useful in diagnosing the problem.* The medical staff and juries expect the patient to be truthful in supplying information so a correct diagnosis may be defined.

Chapter 7: Investigation of an Emergency Department Medical Malpractice Claim

Review of an emergency department claim or a case involving ED care starts with medical records. The emergency department chart is the foundation of any potential or actual ED claim. The attorney should request all the ED records. Copies of the ED record may also be found in the records of subsequent treating physicians. A complete ED chart consists of:

- Face sheet (record of age, address, insurance coverage and so on)
- Triage record
- ED provider examination record – physician, nurse practitioner or physicians assistant
- ED provider orders
- Nursing notes from treatment area – observations, medications, IV fluids, and other treatments
- Diagnostic study results
- Consults from physicians, such as an orthopaedic surgeon who came to the ED to perform a closed reduction of a fracture or a neurosurgeon who evaluated a patient with a head injury
- Consents
- Discharge instructions

The rescue squad records are not often part of the ED chart. However, they should be obtained separately. Clues that the patient came to the ED via rescue squad are found in notations such as

- "BIBA" (brought in by ambulance),
- brought in by "FAS" (first aid squad) or EMS (Emergency Medical Service),
- brought in by (fill in the initials of the specific rescue squad), or
- arrived via MICU (mobile intensive care unit, a highly equipped ambulance designated for critically ill patients).

Determine if the ED medical records are fully electronic or if parts are handwritten. The records could be housed in a lot of different systems and it may be very challenging to get the full record. Carefully review the ED records to be sure all components are there and that there are no time frames that are missing. For example, I reviewed a case in which the allegation was that a patient fell and injured his face in the ED. The patient was in the ED for 12 hours. The hospital's medical records department supplied the triage record. The defense attorney asserted there were no other records for this ED visit. After a judge reviewed my affidavit stating what was missing, he ordered the hospital to produce the records. The case settled shortly after the missing records were provided.

Look for gaps in care, alterations, deletions or omissions. Compare ED records supplied by the hospital with those found within subsequent treating physicians' or hospital records or those supplied to the patient. In short, compare all copies of the ED record to check for inconsistencies or possible alterations. When appropriate, request an audit trail or hire a legal nurse consultant familiar with the software of the ED to further investigate the validity of the ED record.

All hospitals are required to have a control log, which is a registration form that records who came to the ED, and at what time. It records when the patient left the ED and where he or she went (home, back to a nursing home, admission or transfer to another hospital). This log also helps the attorney determine how many other patients were in the ED at the time of the alleged incident. The hospital will block out the other patients' names and data and the confidential information when the log is supplied to the attorney.

Depending on the nature of the allegation, these medical records may be important:

- diagnostic studies such as radiological studies performed during and after the ED care
- a hospital admission after the emergency department evaluation
- outpatient or inpatient treatment post discharge from the hospital
- incident report if an injury occurred within the ED, such as a patient who climbed off a stretcher and fractured his leg

Obtain pertinent hospital ED policies and procedures in effect at the time of the incident. These may be found in a book or may be supplied to the attorney from an electronic file. If the issue was related to triage, obtain the triage manual or policies that were in effect at the time of the care in question. These define the standards of the ED. For example, if the patient presented with a specific complaint such as chest pain, the attorney should request the policies and protocols specific to chest pain. Additionally the triage policy will have details about the different symptoms associated with chest pain that will put a patient into a triage category.

The protocols identify the expected practices. The protocols may be helpful in determining if there was a failure to provide a minimum level of care or if there was substandard care. The standards of care for the patient complaint sometimes will not be in the ED policy and procedures; they will be in the hospital policies and procedures. Since chest pain, for example, could develop in any patient in the ED or within the hospital, there should be standardized approaches to diagnosis and treatment.

Compare the hospital policy and procedures with national standards. The facility must at least meet the national standards. Develop a library of standards. The Emergency Nurses Association publishes standards and provides a mechanism for emergency department nurses to become certified. The American College of Emergency Physicians is the parallel organization.

Identify who documented in the patient's ED chart. Obtain job descriptions of the role and responsibilities of the triage nurse, treatment nurse, and other providers who participated in the patient's care during the time in question. Additionally, the ED may be using unlicensed assistive personnel who were involved in patient care in areas like triage or in the treatment room. Obtain the job description and the policy for use of unlicensed assistive personnel.

Request the personnel files of the staff involved in the patient's care. What did their orientation consist of? Are they certified and by whom? What are their credentials? Were there any disciplinary actions taken against the individual? Some of this information may be obtained directly from the hospital and other details will come out in depositions.

Summary

Care provided in the ED is high risk due to many factors – the unpredictable flow of patients, a vast array of medical conditions, ages and cultures, and the need for astute assessment and diagnostic skills. The ED staff members need to quickly establish rapport with their patients, make decisions, and move the patient through the system while assuring they receive safe, appropriate care. Careful analysis of the liability theories and potential defenses is essential for case selection and for defending ED cases.

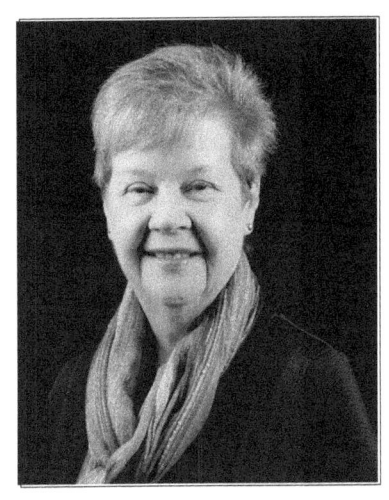

More Resources from Patricia Iyer

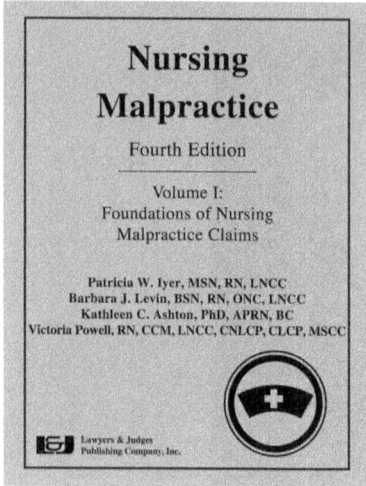
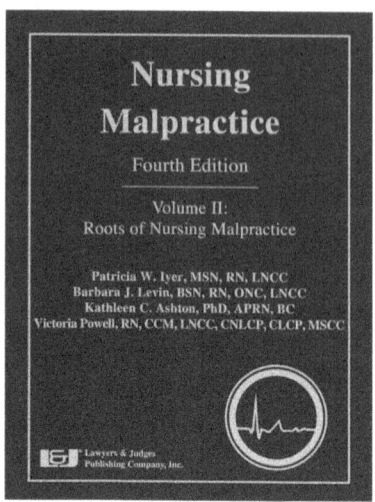

Nursing Malpractice, 4th Edition
Edited by Patricia Iyer, Barbara Levin, Kathleen Ashton, and Victoria Powell

2 volumes in hard cover published in 2011 by Lawyers and Judges Publishing Company

Are you an attorney, legal nurse consultant, expert witness, insurance claims adjuster, healthcare risk manager or clinician?

Nursing Malpractice, Fourth Edition will give you a wealth of information and resources about nursing responsibilities in a wide range of specialties. It covers essential topics that will help you

- Understand nursing roles and practices
- Screen potential nursing malpractice cases
- Evaluate the standard of care

- Use tips and techniques for risk managers for preventing nursing malpractice claims
- Successfully litigate nursing malpractice claims if you are an attorney

A unique blend of attorneys, nurse expert witnesses, legal nurse consultants, physicians, pharmacists, toxicologist, jury consultants, actuaries and legal photographers contributed chapters to this book. This text remains the only one of the market on nursing malpractice that uses such a broad base of expert authors.

Order it today at this link:

www.legalnursebusiness.com

Legal nurse consultants: collect your valuable free ebooks at **www.legalnursebusiness.com**.

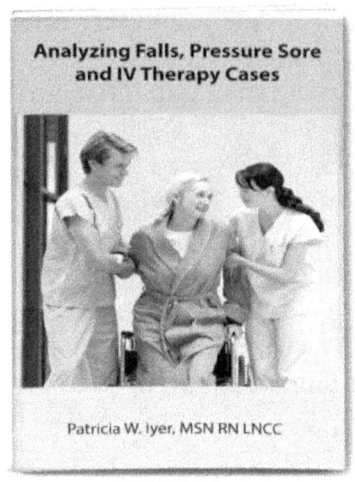

Analyzing Falls, Pressure Sore and IV Therapy Cases

Patricia Iyer MSN RN LNCC
2013
The Pat Iyer Group

Are you a legal nurse consultant, expert witness, attorney or clinician? Falls, pressure sores and IV therapy-related events may lead to high treatment cost, prolonged suffering, and denied reimbursement for hospital care. They may even cause the patient's death.

Healthcare providers are increasingly aware of the clinical and financial risks. Attorneys are seeing an increase in claims related to deviations from the standard of care related to these events.

Analyzing Falls, Pressure Sore and IV Therapy Cases was written to help you understand:

- What causes these events
- What are the clinical results or damages
- How are these problems prevented
- How you can analyze the liability

This text is chock full of practical wisdom, tips, explanations, and guidance for the analysis of these cases. It builds on the author's experiences as an expert witness and legal nurse consultant since 1987.

**Order it today at this link:
www.legalnursebusiness.com**

Book Evaluation Form

Analyzing Emergency Department Medical Malpractice Cases

1. How would you rate the content?
   Excellent ___ Good ___ Average ___ Poor ___

2. Comments about this book:

3. What are your suggestions for future topics?

Please copy this page, complete and fax to 908-806-4511 or mail to The Pat Iyer Group, 11205 Sparkleberry Drive, Fort Myers, FL 33913

Contact Hour Form

Analyzing Emergency Department Medical Malpractice Cases by Patricia Iyer

4 contact hours

Name:

Address:

Street, City, Zip:

1. True/False: A licensed practical nurse may perform the triage role.

2. True/False: The primary goal of triage is to perform a medical screening exam.

3. True/False: Patients is in the waiting area should be periodically reassessed.

To apply for the 4 nursing contact hours, copy and complete this page and send along with a check for $15 written to Taylor College. You may call in a credit card number, if you prefer, to 1-800-743-4006. Please contact Norman Heavens with any questions. Do not send $15 to Patricia Iyer.

Norman Heavens, Taylor College, PO Box 93666
Los Angeles, CA 90093-0666

Consider Writing a Review

Thank you for buying this book. When you enjoy a book, it is a natural desire to tell others about it. Amazon.com provides a way to share your thoughts and I invite you to write a book review. It is easy. Here are tips:

1. After going to the link below on Amazon.com, the first thing you are asked to do is to assign a number of stars to the book you think matches your opinion of the book.

2. Create a title for the review. This can be a simple phrase, like "Awesome guide." If you are not sure what to say, look at the titles of other book reviews.

3. It is easiest to write the book in a word processor and then paste it into Amazon.com Your word processor will pick up typos before your review goes public.

4. Write the review as if you were talking to another person – you are – a person who comes to Amazon.com and is considering buying this book.

5. Include a description of what you found most helpful. Was it an idea, chapter, tip? Share that with the readers.

6. Next you may want to write who you think would most benefit from this book. Is it for beginners? Or is it more appropriate for someone with experience with this topic?

7. What if you have something negative to say about the book? You may always reach me at patriciaiyer@gmail.com to suggest changes in the book.

8. If you include negative feedback in the review, keep a positive perspective rather than attack the author.

Here are some sample phrases:
- While overall the book was good, I would change it by. . .
- I don't think this book is right for. . .
- I would improve this book by. . .

Before you hit save, read everything over one more time.

Authors and readers appreciate book reviews and they get easier to write with time. Go to this link on Amazon.com to write your review. If for any reason it does not work, search for the book title + Iyer and it will show.

Link: http://bit.ly/EDcases

Thank you,
Pat Iyer

www.ingramcontent.com/pod-product-compliance
Lightning Source LLC
Chambersburg PA
CBHW071802170526
45167CB00003B/1141